Atkins Diet

Complete Atkins Diet Guide to Losing Weight and Feeling Amazing!

By Natalie Ray

Table of Contents

Disclaimer

Before you begin any weight loss, exercise or nutritional program, it is recommended that you speak to a qualified health care professional. Professional medical advice should never be disregarded or replaced with the content in this book or anywhere else. Any information or content found within this book is strictly for educational and informational purposes only. Any use of the content within is at your own risk and the author bears no responsibility whatsoever. The author of this book is not affiliated with any medical company, nor does the author provide medical treatment advice in any way. The ideas, views, and opinions expressed in this book are those of the author.

The author assumes no liability for advice or suggestions offered in this book. The author and publisher of this book and the accompanying materials have used their best efforts in preparing this book. The author and publisher make no representation or warranties with respect to the accuracy, applicability, fitness, or completeness of the contents of this book. The information contained in this book is strictly for informational purposes. Therefore, if you wish to apply ideas contained in this book, you are taking full responsibility for your actions.

Introduction

It's a sad but true fact: America is overweight. The worst part of it all is that most aren't doing a single thing about it, and the problem is only getting worse. Did you know that over 50% of the American population is considered overweight? It's a scary thought, isn't it?

More than likely, you've purchased this book because you want to learn more about the Atkins Diet, a diet that has been one of the primary health crazes over the past couple of decades, and how it can help you lose weight. Maybe you've had a health scare or you have simply got tired of looking at yourself in the mirror and wishing you were a few pounds lighter. On the other hand, maybe you don't need to lose weight and you are simply looking for a way to eat healthy and maintain your current weight. Whatever the reason may be, you've decided to go for the Atkins Diet.

Congratulations! for taking charge of your life and choosing the Atkins Diet, one of the most popular, effective and easiest to follow diets today. You are going to need to have some self-control and heavy motivation to stick to the Atkins Diet, as you are going to be limiting the amount of carbs that you eat, which can be really hard for someone used to eating anything that they want without worrying about the effects.

Don't let all of that scare you away, though. The Atkins Diet can be simple to follow and can really help you lose the weight that you are ready to get rid of. Enough of that, though, let's go ahead and delve right into learning more about the Atkins Diet!

About the Atkins Diet

If truth be told right now, you've probably tried diet after diet with little to no success. If you haven't actually been on a diet before, then you must know someone that has. Most diets around require you to count calories and many will require that you avoid foods high in fat. However, there's one particular diet that is very popular and does not require you to do either of those things. In fact, you can eat as much as you'd like of eggs, red meat, bacon, cheese and butter!

As with any other popular diet, and especially with a diet that allows you to eat so many foods that are generally off limits with diets, the Atkins Diet has received much controversy. However, various studies show that the Atkins Diet can help result in weight loss and is actually better than a number of other diets. Not to mention the fact that dieters all over the world are satisfied with the weight loss results that they've achieved with Atkins.

The Atkins Diet is one of the most popular diets out there. It focuses on reducing the intake of carbohydrates while incorporating protein-rich foods. Most of us eat more carbohydrates than anything else in a day, which consists of refined sugar and white flour. In other words, your favorite foods, such as cereal, bread and pasta, contain a large amount of carbohydrates. By limiting your carb intake, you are forcing your body into a state in which it must burn stored fat rather than carbs for fuel.

As already explained, you do need to watch how many carbs are consumed each day; however, there's no need to count calories – which can get a bit mind-numbing when dieting.

So, why do you have to count carbs but not calories? Well, Dr. Atkins, the creator of the Atkins Diet, has performed vigorous research and countless experimentations to come to the conclusion that too many carbohydrates – not too much fat – is actually the main cause of weight gain in individuals. Primarily, this is because when too many carbs enter the body, insulin levels soar triggering fat storage.

How You Lose Weight on the Atkins Diet

At the Atkins Diet focuses on the restriction of carbohydrates. When the body is unable to convert carbs into fuel, it will turn to other methods of creating fuels. With the Atkins Diet, your body will use fat for fuel rather than carbohydrates. Therefore, when consuming little to no carbohydrates, the body's fat storage will thus became its primary source of energy.

In order to really understand how the Atkins Diet helps you lose weight, let's look at how the body creates fuel from sugar. For sugar to be converted into fuel, insulin must be used. Controlling how much sugar is in our blood, insulin makes it possible for the cells in our bodies to turn carbs into glucose. Insulin is secreted to avoid soaring, out of control blood sugar levels. Because insulin is a hormone of storage, sugar that is not converted to fuel will be stored as fat. At the same time, insulin is what keeps the body from efficiently burning stored fat.

According to the Atkins Diet, it is that insulin response that keeps us from losing weight and continuing to add more and more fat to the body. When we have little food, this can be a good thing; however, high-carb and sugar-filled foods will only cause us to accumulate more body fat.

In contract, a low-carb diet will encourage less insulin production. According to the Atkins Diet and various resources online, when your body can maintain a normal insulin level, the body turns to its own fat to convert into fuel. This process results in weight loss. If insulin levels can be kept stable, the body will burn fat and will likely lead to fewer cravings and a suppressed appetite.

So, in a nutshell, the Atkins Diet helps you lose weight by putting you on a very low-carb diet that will help control insulin levels.

The Four Phases of the Atkins Diet

There are four phases in the Atkins Diet: induction, ongoing weight loss, pre-maintenance and maintenance. The duration of each of these phases varies per individual. Atkins now says that you do not have to start with the first phase, but it is recommended since it will give your weight loss efforts a huge boost – even if you can't handle the first phase for the full two weeks that is advised.

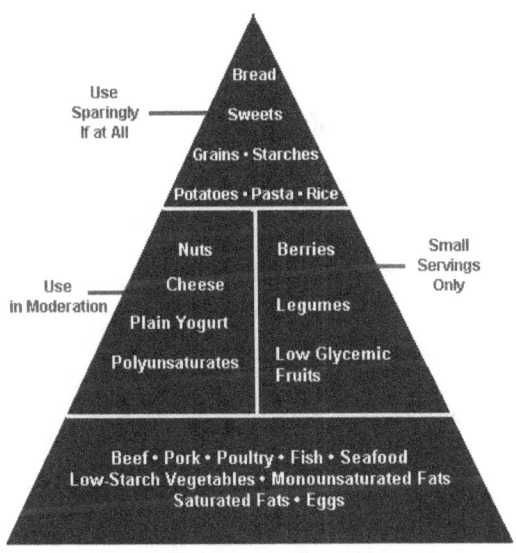

As you move forward with each phase, you will begin to slowly increase your carb intake while avoiding refined sugars and grains. Here's a more in-depth look at each phase, including information on the recommended length of the phase, what you can eat, and the primary goals of that particular phase in your weight loss efforts.

Phase #1 – Induction

This is the most restrictive phase of the diet and it is crucial that you follow this phase to the t. During this phase, which lasts for 14 days, you are allowed to eat very little, if any, carbohydrates. Essentially, you cannot consume more than 20 grams of carbs per day while in the induction phase. The carbs that can be consumed include low-carb, non-starchy vegetables. You can't eat fruits, grains, bread or certain dairy products during the first two weeks of the Atkins Diet.

Ultimately, this first phase is a way to jump-start your weight loss. Although the typical duration is two weeks, you may stay in the first phase for an extra week or so, if you choose, depending on the amount of weight loss you have had towards the end of this phase and your goal weight.

This phase's primary goal is to really get your weight loss journey started with rapid weight loss. When this happens, dieters often feel they are finally doing something right and have a little extra confidence that dieting really can help them lose weight. The induction phase also stabilizes your blood sugar levels, which will minimize, and possibly eliminate, your food cravings. However, keep in mind that you could also experience some mood swings and fatigue from the reduction in carbs and change in your body.

Phase #2 – Ongoing Weight Loss

The second phase gives you the chance to increase the amount of carbs you consume on a daily basis by five grams. You will take this phase week by week, increasing your carb intake by five grains each week. So, it will look like this:

- Week 1: 25 grams of carbs
- Week 2: 30 grams of carbs
- Week 3: 35 grams of carbs
- And so on.

You will continue to slowly increase your intake of carbohydrates until the time when your body hits a plateau and stops losing weight. At this point, you will want to subtract five grams of carbs from your diet each day. This will allow you to maintain your weight. This phase should carry on as long as needed to reach your weight loss goals. Depending on your individual metabolism, you'll consume anywhere from 25 to about 50 carbs per day.

The number of carbohydrates that you can eat while still losing weight is called your Critical Carbohydrate Level for Losing (CCLL) and is one of the primary goals of the Ongoing Weight Loss phase. It has also been developed to help you continue losing weight safely while also learning to consume new foods and limiting your carb intake so that you can still reduce your appetite and cravings.

Phase #3 – Pre-Maintenance

When you hit phase three, your main goal won't be to lose weight, but to maintain it instead. You won't enter this phase until you are within a few pounds of your goal weight – at least 10 pounds. You can increase your carb intake by 10 grams every week as long as you don't start gaining the weight back. Alternatively, you can yourself a nice treat every two or three days by consuming a 20-30 gram carbohydrate item. When you start gaining, you'll need to decrease your carb intake and remain at a lower daily amount.

At this point in the Atkins Diet, the primary goal is to determine how many carbs you can consume on a daily basis without gaining any weight. You will continue to lose weight, but at a much a slower pace, until you reach your final goal. This phase will also help you learn how you can maintain your weight moving forward.

Phase #4 – Lifetime Maintenance

The fourth and final phase of the Atkins Diet still limits your carbohydrate intake, but gives you a larger variety of foods to select from. This phase will help you ensure that the pounds you have lost do not come back while giving you more freedom when it comes to what you eat.

You will have to ensure you keep the bad, refined carbs out of your diet and only take in healthy carbs. As long as you pull together everything that you have learned thus far while on the Atkins Diet, you should have no problem successfully keeping your weight off since you know now your body's limit when it comes to carbohydrates. Most people will find that the right amount of carbs is between 75 and 100 grams of carbs per day.

Ultimately, at this point in time, you've reached your goal weight and are ready to move forward with your life in a new, improved and sexy body!

Pros and Cons of the Atkins Diet

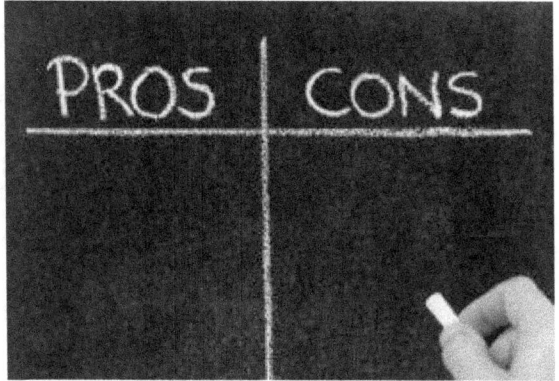

Pros:

- **The ability to eat usually forbidden foods.** More often than not, when you go on a diet, you aren't permitted to eat butter, steak and other foods with high fat counts. With the Atkins Diet, you can. However, don't concentrate on one type of fat and you should never forget your

Omega-3 fatty acids and olive oil.

- **Easy to start, easy to stick to.**

  Ultimately, the Atkins Diet is pretty easy and straightforward. While the induction phase may be a bit of a stretch when it comes to "easy", for the most part, the Atkins Diet is one of the easiest diets to follow without putting a whole lot of time, energy and thought into what you are eating, especially after you learn the best foods to eat.

- **Teaches weight maintenance.** One of the hardest things to learn is how to maintain your weight once you do lose it. The Atkins Diet helps you learn how many carbs you can consume each day without gaining weight. This occurs through a gradual increase of carbs on a weekly basis until you reach the amount of carbs that you can safely eat without gaining a pound.

- **Prevents disease.** When you lower the amount of carbs you are putting in your body, you are ultimately reducing the production of insulin, which helps to prevent certain diseases, particularly diabetes.

Cons:

- **Requires counting.** Because the Atkins Diet centers around the amount of carbohydrates you are consuming, you'll be counting your carbs all the time. This can get really boring and old after a while, but it's worth it if you're losing weight.

- **Induction Phase.** It's no walk in the park, but it really helps give your body that extra kick in the butt it needs to get started losing weight. Remember, this phase is not the entire diet, and you will be able to introduce new foods to your diet as you move forward into the Atkins Diet.

- **Carb crash.** It's possible for your body to "crash" after a few days into the Atkins Diet, especially if you are doing the

Induction phase. You just need to eat a few more carbs, but don't overdo it. Don't let the feeling that you had when you crashed keep you from moving forward onto bigger (or I guess smaller since you'll be losing weight) and better things.

- **Determining carb levels.** Many dieters look away from the Atkins Diet because of the whole counting carbs aspect and finding the right level of carbohydrates that will keep you from gaining weight. Adding five grams of carbs per week can be a bit tedious and difficult to do.

- **Minor side effects.** While they aren't huge problems, there are a few side effects that can be experienced with the Atkins Diet including, but not limited to bad breath, constipation, fatigue, headaches, brain fog, muscle cramps, and mood swings.

Top Mistakes Made by Atkins Dieters

As with any diet, there are mistakes to be made by the dieter. It's part of life. However, as I tell you the most common mistakes made by those on the Atkins Diet, I'm also going to give you a few hints as to what you can do to maybe keep from making the mistake or make the impact of the mistake much less dramatic.

1. **Stop dieting after the induction phase because of less weight loss.** During the induction phase, because the diet is so incredibly restrictive, you will lose a decent amount of weight. In fact, you could lose five pounds a week or more,

depending on your body and your exercise regimen. Once you move onto the next phase, you will begin eating more carbs and your weight loss will slow down, but it will not just abruptly stop. Don't let the fact that you may only lose a pound or two one week get you down so much that you stop dieting. The pounds will continue to fall off, but the Atkins Diet, just as any other diet, is no miracle overnight weight loss program. Have patience, remain confident and stay on track with the Atkins Diet and you'll continue to lose those unwanted pounds.

2. **Not eliminating caffeine from the diet.** Because so many of us are addicted to

soft drinks, it's hard to get rid of them cold turkey when you start on the Atkins Diet. Instead, try weaning yourself from your favorite soda pop before you actually start the Atkins Diet. This will help you adjust before you get started on the actual diet and you probably won't have a problem giving them up. If nothing else, and while it is most definitely not recommended, you could limit yourself to one soda every few days or a little bit of a sip each day. Again, this isn't recommended but it may keep you balanced enough to where you can continue your diet.

3. **Eating too much cheese.** Just because you can eat cheese while on the Atkins

Diet doesn't mean you can overdo it. You need to limit yourself to approximately four ounces of cheese per day because cheese does have a small amount of carbohydrates.

4. **Not eating enough vegetables.** You need to eat plenty of vegetables when on the Atkins Diet, especially since it is the primary source of food during the induction phase. The problem is that most people will eat more meat than vegetables, and the body needs nutrients and vitamins from those veggies.

5. **Eating too much.** While you don't need to count your calories while on the Atkins

Diet, it doesn't mean that calories aren't important. With a low-carb diet such as the Atkins Diet, your hunger and cravings will be suppressed, which means you can consume fewer calories without getting those hunger pains. Many dieters believe that they can just keep eating and eating without it causing any problems with their weight loss goals. Truth be told, it is possible to eat too much, even while on the Atkins Diet. You don't necessarily have to count your calories, but don't overstuff. Stop eating when you feel comfortable and only eat when you feel hungry.

6. **Adding a few carbs here and there.** So, you've started your Atkins Diet. You've dropped several pounds and you're feeling great. You aren't having cravings between meals and you have a ton of energy. You think that it'll be okay to have a piece of toast with your breakfast one morning. It's just once and you still feel great. Then you think you will have a small bowl of ice cream. You're still shedding the weight so a little sugar in your tea won't do much harm either, right? You end up going over your carb limit. You're now having cravings, gaining a few pounds and back to where you started – having problems breaking the consumption of carbs. You feel hungrier

so you eat a few more carbs. It may not happen like this for you, but the fact is that it happens. You will probably need to start all the way over with the Atkins Diet. It's a tough cycle to break, but it can be done with time, patience, dedication, motivation and effort.

7. **Not exercising.** Because you will see success of weight loss on the Atkins Diet at first without exercising, you may think that you don't need to perform any physical activity. However, it is important to exercise, as it also helps lower insulin resistance, not to mention the fact that exercise is just healthy for your body overall. If you aren't used to exercising,

then just take things slow, but don't omit it from your weight loss program completely. You will find that exercise will help you speed up your weight loss and get in shape.

Atkins Diet Grocery Shopping List

When you first start yourself on the Atkins Diet, it can be difficult heading off to the grocery store and not having the slightest clue as to what to purchase. To help you get started, here's a list of low-carb products that you can pick up at the grocery store:

- Cucumber
- Celery
- Broccoli
- Asparagus
- Green beans

- Peppers (red, yellow and green)
- Spinach
- Cabbage
- Cauliflower
- Snow Peas

- Salad greens

- Tomatoes

- Full-fat

  dressings

- Cheese

- Eggs

- Fish

- Shellfish

- Tuna (check

  labels on

  canned tuna)

- Chicken

- Pork

- Unprocessed

  meat

- Bacon

- Sausage

- Strawberries

- Blueberries

- Raspberries

- Blackberries

- Cantaloupe

- Peaches

- Squash

- Avocadoes

- Melon

- Nuts –

  almonds,

  macadamia,

  etc.

- Extra virgin

  and unrefined

oils – olive, sesame and coconut, peanut

If you decide to purchase something not on the above list, then that's fine. Don't think that you need to stick to this list. However, be sure to read the food label and you'll want to pay particular attention to – yes, you guessed it – the amount of carbohydrates that the product contains. You'll need to pay extra special attention to the carb amount during the first two weeks of your diet since you can only have 20 carbs maximum per day.

Permitted Beverages on the Atkins Diet

Here's a look at the beverages that can be consumed while following the Atkins Diet:

- Caffeine-free tea
- Caffeine-free diet soft drinks
- Still or sparkling water
- Decaffeinated coffee
- Club soda
- Lime or lemon juice
- Cream – no milk
- Bouillon

You can use artificial sweeteners, such as Equal, Splenda or Sweet 'n' Low. If you prefer to go natural, Stevia is fine as well.

When it comes to water, it is important to drink about six to eight glasses of water per day. This helps keep you fully hydrated while on the Atkins Diet. After the Induction phase, you can add lemon, lime and tomato juice into your diet, but be careful to watch carbohydrate counts.

Basically, if you want to drink anything other than what has been mentioned here, you will want to check the nutritional label on the beverage closely and verify that you won't be going over your daily carbohydrate count if you drink it. Remember, the amount of carbohydrates that you consume each day is the most important thing when on the Atkins Diet – a few extra carbs can really hurt the diet in the long-run.

Foods to Eat by Phase

Curious about what foods you can eat during each phase of the Atkins Diet? Here's a brief look to help you understand what you can and can't have during each of the four phases of the low-carb diet program.

Induction Phase Foods

Basically, your protein is going to come from chicken, tuna, salmon, turkey, beef, bacon, sausage, pork, eggs, etc. You will need to avoid processed meats, such as lunch meat. In addition, avoid meats with breaded crusts. Although there is no limit on your fat intake when on the Atkins Diet, it is important not to overdo it. Opt for healthy fats, such as avocadoes, olive oil and the like. You cannot have milk or yogurt, but you can have full-fat cream cheese, butter and sour cream.

During the induction phase, you can only have 20 carbs and those carbs will come from non-starchy veggies, such as celery, lettuce, peppers, broccoli, spinach, eggplant, cauliflower, asparagus, etc. You'll want to avoid pasta, carrots, corn, potatoes and grains.

Ongoing Weight Loss Phase Foods

When you reach this phase, you'll get to start increasing your carbs, which means you'll be able to consume a larger variety of food. Remember, it's only five grams of carbs each week, so you won't be able to do too much at once. However, you can start consuming more dairy products, nuts, berries, fruits, starchy veggies, grains, legumes and even alcohol, if you desire. Just don't forget to keep track of those carbs!

Pre-Maintenance and Maintenance Phase Foods

Basically, any and all of the aforementioned foods are permitted during these two phases. These phases are more individualized and customized than the initial two phases, so it's going to vary from one person to the next when it comes to how many carbs can be consumed each day. You'll have to find your own personal carb level for a steady and healthy weight.

Atkins Daily Food Menu and Cooking Recipes

Here's a look at what a typically day on the Atkins Diet might look like:

Breakfast: A mix of sausage and scrambled eggs, with an approved beverage.

Snack: Atkins Diet granola bar.

Lunch: Grilled chicken on salad greens with dressing, onions, olives and bean sprouts, along with a permitted beverage.

Snack: String cheese and avocadoes.

Dinner: Arugula salad with cucumbers and cherry tomatoes, asparagus, baked salmon steak and an approved beverage.

Sample Cooking Recipes for Each Meal

To help you get started cooking low-carb meals for yourself, here are a few cooking recipes for each meal.

Breakfast Low-Carb Pancakes

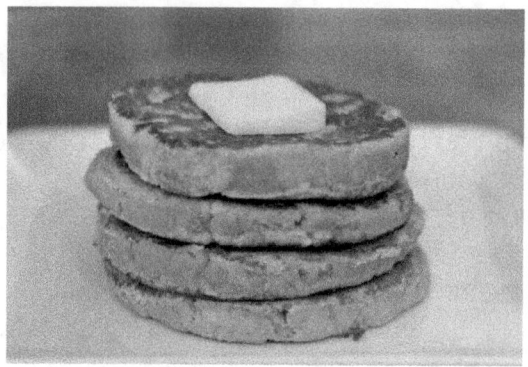

- 2 eggs

- 1 cup of almond meal (instead of white flour)

- ¼ cup of water

- 2 tablespoons of olive oil

- ¼ teaspoon of salt

- 1 tablespoon of artificial sweetener (no sugar!)

Mix together and cook just as you would any other type of pancake. Serve with sugar-free maple syrup, strawberry topping or any other form of topping that consists of low carbs.

*Only one gram of carbohydrates per 4-inch pancake.

Old-Fashioned Meat Loaf

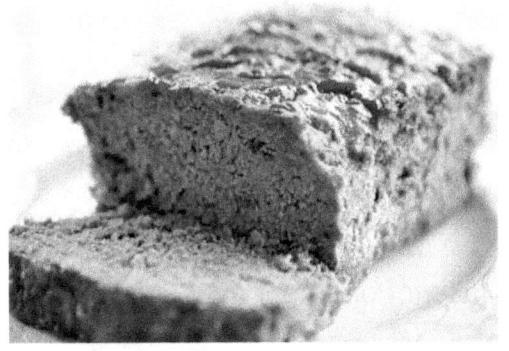

- Two pounds of ground meat (the leaner the better)
- 1 cup of TVP (can be omitted)
- 2 garlic cloves, minced (or 1 tsp of garlic powder)
- ¼ cup onion, finely chopped

- 1 teaspoon dried sage

- 1 teaspoon dried thyme

- 1 teaspoon dry mustard powder

- 2 teaspoons of salt

- 2 tablespoons of Worcestershire sauce

- 1 egg

- ¼ cup of milk or water

Mix everything together in a large bowl. You can bake in one large loaf pan or several smaller ones. Bake for one hour at 350 degrees. Add a sugar-free picante sauce over the top about 15 minutes prior to the meat loaf being done.

*One serving has just two grams of carbohydrates.

Broccoli and Bacon Salad

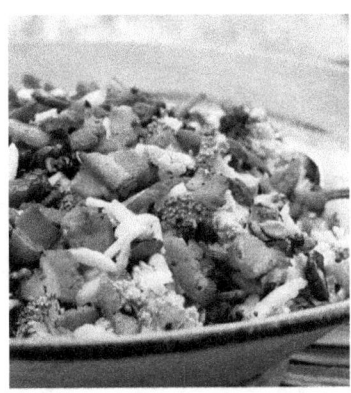

- 5 cups of chopped steams and flowerettes of broccoli

- ½ pound of bacon (cooked crisp, drained of grease/fat and chopped)

- ¼ cup of onion, finely chopped

- ¾ cup of mayo

- 1 ½ tablespoons of lemon juice (or to taste)

- 1 tablespoon of sugar substitute (zero-card, preferably)

- ¼ cup of sunflower seeds

- 2 tablespoons of dried currants

- Salt and pepper (to taste)

Boil or microwave broccoli for about two minutes. It should soften, but still be crunchy. Cool in a bowl of ice water or run it under cold tap water. Mix the lemon juice, mayo, sweetener and a little bit of salt and pepper in a bowl to make your dressing. Add in the dried currants and finely chopped onions. Mix the dressing in a bowl with the broccoli and remaining ingredients. You can save a small amount of bacon and sunflower seeds to sprinkle on the top, if you'd like.

*One serving contains three grams of carbohydrates.

Easy Oven-Roasted Asparagus

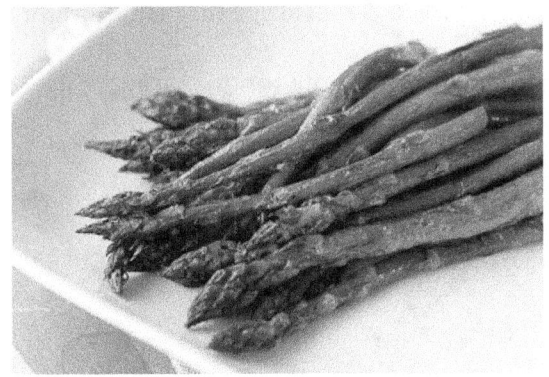

- Asparagus

- One teaspoon of olive oil per six spears of
  asparagus

- Salt and pepper, along with choice herbs

- Few drops of lemon or lime juice
  (optional)

Heat the oven to 425 degrees (or you can heat
the grill, if you prefer). Prepare the asparagus for
cooking by breaking off the ends or any other
way you are comfortable with. Place spears on

cookie sheet and drizzle oil over the top of the spears. Sprinkle salt, pepper, herbs and lemon or lime juice. Bake until tender, about 5 to 10 minutes.

*One 5-7-inch long asparagus spear contains .3 grams of carbohydrates.

Eating Out While on the Atkins Diet

Love eating out? Of course you do – almost everyone does. However, heading out to your favorite restaurant for dinner can have some dire consequences if you aren't careful. Luckily, there are a few things that you can do to ensure you stick to your Atkins Diet and still enjoy going out to eat every once in a while.

Whether your favorite food is Chinese, Mexican or Italian, as long as you stick to a few small guidelines, you can eat out without feeling guilty! Keep reading to find out these guidelines, as well as a few tips to help you along the way, and some great food items that are on some of your favorite fast food restaurant menus. I'll even help you determine low-carb eating solutions for Chinese, Italian and Mexican restaurants.

General Eating Out Tips

Before we just delve into foods that you can eat when dining out, let's look at a few basic principles.

1. Order foods with plenty of protein and fiber.

2. Avoid trans fat.

3. Choose leafy greens.

4. Avoid refined sugars.

5. Opt for grilled chicken instead of crispy chicken.

6. Always do away with the bun/bread on burgers and sandwiches.

7. Don't be afraid to take your own spices/dressing to the restaurant.

8. Always start your meal with a healthy salad. (Low carbs, high fiber)

9. Ask for substitutions. Usually, to keep your service, restaurants will accommodate your request.

Eating Out at McDonald's

As the largest fast food chain worldwide, McDonald's is a hard habit to break when you go on a diet. When ordering a burger from McDonald's, you will want to order it without the bun – or take the bun off when you get it. This removes the carbs. The cheese and vegetables will have about one gram of carbohydrates each and Big Mac sauce and ketchup will have about two grams.

If you opt for chicken or fish, be careful because you will get a decent amount of carbs, depending on how it's cooked. For example, grilled chicken only has a couple of grams of carbs while the Filet-o-Fish and crispy chicken has 9-10 grams of carbs each.

If you opt for salad, you'll only get about three grams of carbs with the side salad – and plenty of nutrition and greens! Salad with grilled chicken nets about 9 grams of carbs and crispy chicken salads have as much as 38 carbs. Stick to Caesar Salads and Bacon Ranch Salads with GRILLED chicken to limit your carb intake.

Don't even think about eating McNuggets, French fries or any type of dessert from McDonald's. You'll totally botch your diet if you do.

Checkout McDonald's website for nutritional information ahead of time. It allows you to view any item on their menu and click/un-click certain parts of that item, such as the bun, to see the amount of carbs.

Eating Out at Burger King

The same advice goes for Burger King as it did for McDonald's. Eat without the bun. Opt for grilled chicken sandwiches, as they'll only have a few grams of carbs. In fact, the only sensible low-carb Atkins-approved chicken sandwich at Burger King is the Tendergrill Chicken Sandwich with 3 grams of carbs – without the bun. The Tendergrill is the only logical salad choice, as well, at 8 grams.

Eating Out at Subway

Obviously, Subway is healthier than McDonald's and Burger King, but do they have anything for low-carb, Atkins Diet followers? Unfortunately, because the tortillas and bread have so many carbs, there are not many options at Subway when on the Atkins Diet. You are going to have to opt for salads, netting about 10 grams of carbs. Choose your dressing wisely though – the oil and vinegar has zero carbs while the red wine vinaigrette has about 17 carbs.

Eating Out at Chinese Restaurants

When eating out at a Chinese restaurant, you must be careful or you'll quickly consume too many carbs. You will want to avoid rice, noodles, wontons, egg rolls and breaded meats. Your best bets are going to be stir-fried dishes, steamed foods, clear and thin soups and walnut chicken. If you choose a meat and vegetable combination or any other dish, limit the sauce, especially if it is thick and spicy, as this means more starch and sugar. If you aren't careful, you could take in about seven grams of carbohydrates with just one tablespoon of cornstarch. If all else fails, ask for the sauce to be on the side.

Eating Out at Mexican Restaurants

While there are plenty of items to avoid at a Mexican restaurant, there's also plenty that is safe for you. You'll want to skip the chips and salsa; although, I know, they look so appetizing. You can, however, have the guacamole with your entrée. Speaking of your entrée, you'll want to stick to a few items, such as grilled meats and seafood. You can have fajitas and tostado salads, but skill the tortillas and shell. If you want to opt for a stew/soup dish, have the chili verde.

Ultimately, at a Mexican restaurant, here's what you want to avoid: tacos, tortillas, burritos, nachos, taquitos, enchiladas, quesadillas, tamales, flautas, and chimichangas. The reason these are on the avoid list is because of the outside shell, so if you want to order just the filling of a chimichanga, go right ahead.

Eating Out at Italian Restaurants

Sure, Italian food consists of pizza, pasta and delicious bread – all of which are full of carbohydrates – but that doesn't mean that there aren't some decent, low-carb dishes that you can savor while on the Atkins Diet. When it comes to appetizers, stick to seafood, meats and veggies.

If you want soup, you'll want to stick to the thinner soups, such as seafood soups, Stracciatelle and vegetable soups. Obviously, a salad is a fine choice while on Atkins, but avoid the croutons. The variety of seafood and meats on the menu will be fine, as long as you steer

clear of the breaded meats.

How to Accelerate Weight Loss

It's great that you've decided to try the Atkins Diet to lose weight, but you honestly need to do more than just diet. While you will lose weight dieting alone, you could increase the amount of weight that you lose and speed up the pounds shedding off if you add an exercise regimen into your weight loss program.

The best way to reach your goal weight is to make lifestyle changes, which includes the Atkins Diet and sweating it out at the gym or at home on a regular basis. Here are some tips to help you speed up the weight loss process and simply stay on top of things:

1. **Use your scale.** Don't weight yourself every single day. Instead, only weigh in about once per week. Try to make it on the same day and at the same time. The best time to weigh yourself is first thing in the morning before you have put anything in your body and your digestive system is clean.

2. **Exercise regularly.** To speed up weight loss now and to keep the weight off in the future, it's important to exercise. You should perform around 2-3 hours per week of moderate intensity aerobic exercise or half of that of vigorous intensity. In addition, you should spend two days or more focusing on strength

training each muscle group.

3. **Make sure you have plenty of support around you.** It can be hard to stick to a diet and exercise activity if you don't have support of family and friends. In some cases, many dieters find that support will actually help speed up the weight loss process because they stay on track.

4. **Fight your food cravings.** Giving into your food cravings is a definite way to slow down the process of losing weight. Not only will you eat more than you should, but you will also start gaining your weight back. You will want to make sure that when you start on the Atkins Diet that

you remove all prohibited foods from your home (soda, candy, ice cream, etc.). Fill your home with the healthy, low-carb foods that you can have.

5. **Do not starve yourself.** This is the quickest way to hurt yourself and to do damage to your dieting efforts. You aren't going to be doing your body any good starving it. Did you know that when you skip meals it can actually cause you to have excessive hunger pains? We all know hunger pains only lead to trouble!

6. **Beware of binge eating.** When you get stressed out or have a lot on your plate, it is possible that you will begin to binge eat,

which is when you eat a large amount of food without a short period of time. This will most definitely harm your weight loss process. Instead of perusing the fridge for carbs, head out for a brisk walk or go to the gym to get your mind on something else.

7. **Consider a diet buddy.** Sometimes it can be heard to diet and exercise alone. If you have someone that wants to lose weight as much as you, then it can actually be fun to exercise. You can share motivational tips and recipes while keeping each other on track.

Remember, you are responsible for your weight loss. No one and nothing else. If you can't put in the time and effort to shed those unwanted pounds, then you aren't going to get that slim, sexy body that you've always dreamed of. Set yourself some goals and stick to your diet and exercise regimen. It's the only way to lose weight.

How to Keep the Weight Off

Did you know that probably about 90 percent of all dieters that lose weight while on a diet regain that weight or at least a portion of that weight within a year's time? You don't want to be in that 90 percent.

Aside from sticking to the maintenance phase of the Atkins Diet, there are plenty of other ways that you can help yourself keep the weight off. Here are some tips on how to keep the weight off:

- Exercise on a daily basis or at least as often as possible. Use every opportunity you have to exercise, even if it's just 15 minutes.

- Make sure resistance training is part of your exercise workout. This will help you maintain muscle mass.

- Don't start stuffing your face with carbs. You've worked so hard to get to where you are, and you did that by eating fewer carbs each day. Don't damage everything you've done so far by getting addicted to carbs again.

- Reduce fried and refined foods, as these are empty calories.

- Stay hydrated. Water ensures that your metabolism is strong and continues to burn calories efficiently.

- Keep your stress levels as stable as possible. When you become stressed, cortisol is produced raising insulin resistance and encouraging storage of fat.

- Make sure to get as much sleep as possible. Adults need about eight hours of sleep per night.

- Continue to weigh yourself on a regular basis so that if you do start to gain weight, you catch it early on and can get those pounds off quickly.

Exercise is most definitely going to be one of the best ways to keep the weight off after you lose it. There are various programs out there, such as Zumba and CrossFit, so that you don't just head out to the gym and get on a boring treadmill. Exercise can become tedious after a while if you don't shake things up a bit. Taking a dance class or swimming a few laps around the pool can help keep things fresh so that you aren't always at the gym working out. Also, try amping up your workouts. If you've been walking for 30 minutes, try adding another 30 minutes to that or turning your walk into a jog.

You've lost the weight and now all you have to do is keep it off. If you continue eating healthy and exercising regularly, you'll find that it's quite easy to keep the weight off and maintain a tone body.

Conclusion

The Atkins Diet has been a diet that people have used to lose weight for years. The primary obstacle that dieters face when on the Atkins Diet is how to avoid the bad habits and pitfalls that caused them to be overweight to begin with. By establishing a healthy diet plan and habits, such as low-carb eating and no skipping of meals, while also finding ways to deal with emotional issues (stress) that could possibly influence your eating habits, you will be well on your way to a healthier, better-feeling and more confident you!

Keep in mind, it will get easier over time because your strategies to keep the pounds off will eventually become like second nature to you and

require little to no effort on your part. Put in the
time and you will reap the benefits!

Best wishes,

-Natalie Ray

www.ingramcontent.com/pod-product-compliance
Lightning Source LLC
Chambersburg PA
CBHW070307290526
45791CB00003B/1099